'Davida Hartman's book *Beating Anxiety* is a beautifully written, simple and concise insight into anxiety and autism. Page by page, she demystifies anxiety and provides strategies and techniques to give young people the confidence and tools to overcome worries and stresses that prevent them from enjoying life. Its accessibility to children and positivity is a perfect antidote to the monster that anxiety can be to us all.'

– Paula Rudkins, Children's Service Manager, Enable Ireland

'An enormously valuable and accessible resource for people on the autism spectrum who are experiencing anxiety. Hartman eloquently strikes the right balance with her tips to tackle anxiety from a physical, behavioural and cognitive perspective, while providing essential psychoeducation around anxiety and emotions in general. This is an empowering "must-read" for anyone with ASD.'

– Roisin Doyle, Cognitive Behavioural Psychotherapist,
Stillorgan Medical Centre

'Davida Hartman superbly captures practical tools and strategies to beat stress and anxiety and in turn generate calm and relaxation. Davida's skills as a clinician shine through on every page and the illustrations offer the parent, child and therapists relevant evidence-based interventions.'

– Dr Eddie Murphy, clinical psychologist and author

BEATING ANXIETY

BEATING ANXIETY

What Young People on the Autism Spectrum Need to Know

Davida Hartman

Illustrated by Kate Brangan

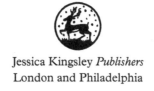

Jessica Kingsley *Publishers*
London and Philadelphia

First published in 2017
by Jessica Kingsley Publishers
73 Collier Street
London N1 9BE, UK
and
400 Market Street, Suite 400
Philadelphia, PA 19106, USA

www.jkp.com

Copyright © Davida Hartman 2017
Illustrations copyright © Kate Brangan 2017

Front cover image source: Kate Brangan

Library of Congress Cataloging in Publication Data
Names: Hartman, Davida, author.
Title: Beating anxiety : what young people on the autism spectrum need to
    know / Davida Hartman.
Description: Philadelphia : Jessica Kingsley Publishers, [2017] | Audience:
    Age: 8-15. | Includes bibliographical references and index.
Identifiers: LCCN 2016046970 (print) | LCCN 2016057721 (ebook) | ISBN
    9781785920752 (alk. paper) | ISBN 9781784503352 (ebook)
Subjects: LCSH: Anxiety in children--Juvenile literature. | Autistic
    children--Juvenile literature.
Classification: LCC BF723.A5 H37 2017 (print) | LCC BF723.A5 (ebook) | DDC
    155.4/1246--dc23
LC record available at https://lccn.loc.gov/2016046970

British Library Cataloguing in Publication Data
A CIP catalogue record for this book is available from the British Library

ISBN 978 1 78592 075 2
eISBN 978 1 78450 335 2

Printed and bound in Great Britain

For Alex

CONTENTS

INTRODUCTION   11

ANXIETY AND THE AUTISM SPECTRUM

1. ANXIETY   19

2. ANXIETY AND THE AUTISM SPECTRUM   27

THINGS YOU CAN DO TO BEAT ANXIETY

Get to Know You   35

Change What You Can   39

Learn About Emotions (and Try Not to Avoid Them)   42

Express Your Emotions   46

Look After Your Body   48

Learn How to Deep Breathe   53

Face Your Fears   56

Give Anxiety a Name and a Shape   59

Talk Back to Anxiety   61

Throw Away Anxiety   64

Think Positive Thoughts   66

Imagine Relaxing Pictures   69

Put Your Worries to the Test   73

Be Mindful   76

Meditate   79

Daily Relaxing Time   82

Whole Body Relaxation   84

Three Ways Your Hands and Arms Can Help You Relax   86

Have a Signal   88

Dealing with Sensory Overload   91

Dealing with Panic Attacks   94

Practise Being Grateful   96

EXTRA INFORMATION FOR ADULTS

INFORMATION FOR PARENTS AND PROFESSIONALS   *101*

RECOMMENDED READING AND RESOURCES FOR
PARENTS AND PROFESSIONALS   *108*

INTRODUCTION

If you are reading this book, you probably have something called autism or Asperger syndrome. Or, as I will call it from now on, you are **on the autism spectrum**. There are lots of great things about being on the autism spectrum, many of which you will read about in this book.

You probably also deal with something called **anxiety**. Anxiety is one of the not so great things about being on the autism spectrum.

Anxiety is when you are feeling really worried or afraid of something that you think might happen in the future.

Anxiety affects people differently. It might make you:

- Worry all day about lots of different things

- Be intensely afraid of just one or two things

- Feel anxious when you are around other people

- Find it even harder than normal to deal with sensory information (sounds, sights, noises, tastes, touch and smells)

- Get things called panic attacks (when you get so overwhelmed by anxiety that you feel as if you can't breathe or think or move)

- Have meltdowns

- Stay awake at night worrying about things that might happen in the future

- Get stomach or head aches

- Become very focused on keeping everything in your life exactly the same

- Become very focused on having everything in your life happen at exactly the same time each day

If any of this sounds familiar to you, don't worry! This book is full of tactics or strategies that will help you learn to:

- Calm your body and mind

- Live a calmer and happier life

- Cope with normal, day-to-day anxiety

- Prevent unhealthy anxiety building up

- Prevent meltdowns and panic attacks

- Deal with meltdowns and panic attacks when they do happen

- Break the 'loop of worry', where one fear leads to another

- Be more resilient (able to cope with difficult things that might happen in the future)

- Be mentally fit (just like how exercising gets your body physically fit)

What is brilliant about the tactics in this book is that they all work! But I'm not going to lie to you: practising them might not be easy at first. You might find some of them boring. You might try a few things (like closing your eyes and taking deep breaths) that make you feel giggly or a bit uncomfortable. You might feel stressed when you do them at first (which is weird since they are supposed to reduce stress!). But remember that they are NEW. And new can be difficult, especially when you are on the autism spectrum. If you are finding some of the tactics difficult, don't give up. You might not be used to them yet. You might just need a bit of extra help with them. Everyone is different and will like different tactics better than others.

A LESSON FROM TEMPLE GRANDIN
ABOUT TRYING NEW THINGS

Temple Grandin is a famous and very clever woman on the autism spectrum. She travels all over the world talking to big groups of people about what it is like to have autism and about all of her amazing achievements. Lots of people on the autism spectrum don't like new things, and Temple says she is one of these people. At one of her talks, she told everyone a story about the first time she went on a rollercoaster. She said that she really didn't like it. But the problem was that she didn't know whether she didn't like it because it was NEW or for some other reason. So you know what she did? She went on the rollercoaster a few more times, *just to make sure*. Turned out she really didn't like rollercoasters! Temple says that she uses this tactic (trying new things a few times) with everything in her life. And while she probably won't go on a rollercoaster ever again, there are lots of other things in her life that she now loves, all because she **kept trying**.

HOW YOU CAN USE THIS BOOK

1. Read it on your own or with another person.

2. Pick a tactic to work on (it might be a good idea to pick an easy one first).

3. Put a reminder of the tactic somewhere obvious that you pass by every day (maybe on your bedroom wall or on the fridge).

4. Practise it every day for about a month.

5. Get your family or friends involved.

6. At the end of the month, answer these questions: Is this tactic helping? Do I feel more relaxed or calm after doing it? Do I like it? Do I want to keep doing it?

7. If the tactic is helping to reduce anxiety, keep doing it every day or when you need it. Then pick another tactic to try.

8. If the tactic *isn't* working at the moment, try a new one.

9. Of course, you don't have to choose just one tactic. Try as many as you like!

CREATING A HABIT

When you do something every day it eventually becomes a HABIT. When something is a habit it takes a lot less effort to do. Sometimes we are not even aware that we are doing it. When you practise these tactics every day at around the same time, you are on your way to turning them into healthy habits to last a lifetime.

ANXIETY AND THE AUTISM SPECTRUM

ANANXIETY

1

There are lots of different words for anxiety, like stress, nerves, fears, panic, worries, freaking out, jumpiness, being afraid or agitation. It can feel different at different times. Sometimes it can feel like anger. Sometimes it can make you feel upset, sad, overwhelmed or irritable.

The first thing you need to know about anxiety is that it is NORMAL. Everyone feels anxiety some of the time. In fact, a LITTLE bit of anxiety is a good thing. It helps prepare our bodies for danger. It helps us get things done that need to get done (like study for a big exam). It helps our memory and focus (for example, *during* that big exam). Some people even say that a little bit of stress as a child is a good thing because it makes us stronger and more able to cope with bad stuff that might happen when we are adults.

The problem is that while a little bit of anxiety is normal or can even be a good thing, TOO MUCH anxiety is like your worst enemy. If your brain was a computer, too much anxiety would be like a computer virus taking over and stopping it working properly. Too much anxiety makes you more likely to get sick. It feels terrible. It can stop you achieving things that you want to in life. It is bad for your relationships with other people. It can make you worry about things that aren't real. Because of it, you miss out on a lot of amazing and wonderful things. When you are very anxious you can't think properly. You can't use your words properly or understand fully what people say to you. You get clumsy and bump into things. It is also very hard to make good decisions.

Here is a picture with some of the kinds of THOUGHTS people have when they are anxious or stressed. Do you ever think thoughts like these?

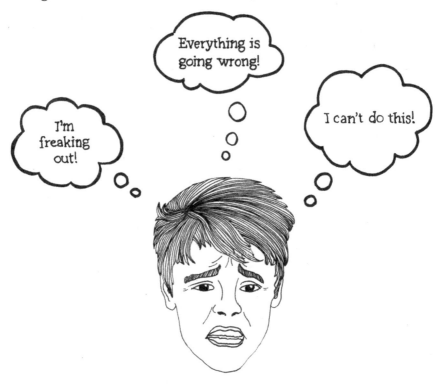

Here is a picture of some of the ways that anxiety can LOOK or FEEL in your body. Do you ever feel any of these?

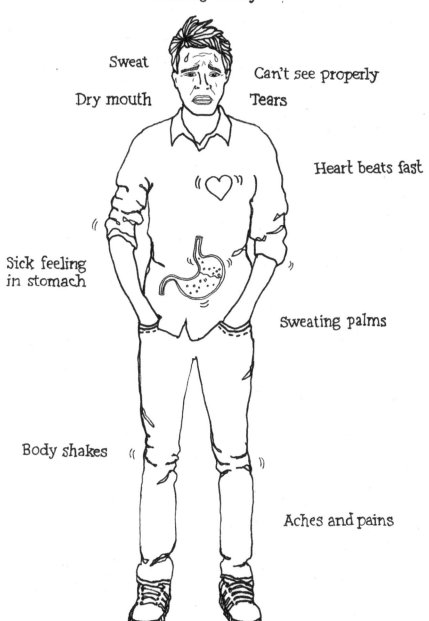

Difficulty thinking clearly

Sweat

Dry mouth

Can't see properly

Tears

Heart beats fast

Sick feeling in stomach

Sweating palms

Body shakes

Aches and pains

Here are some pictures of how people sometimes ACT or BEHAVE when they feel anxious.

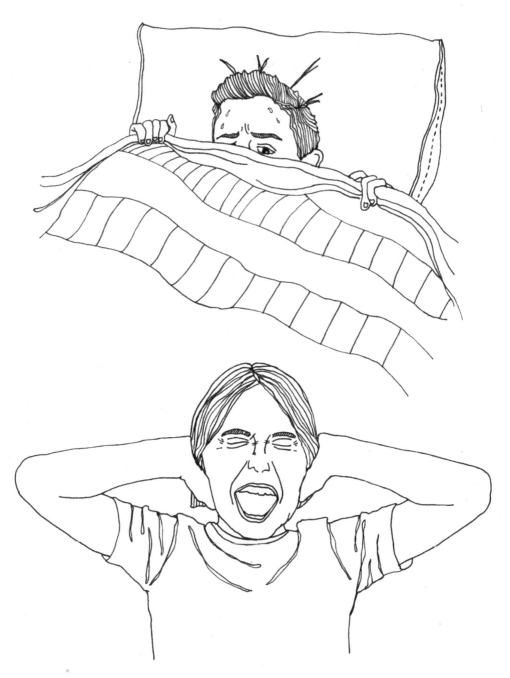

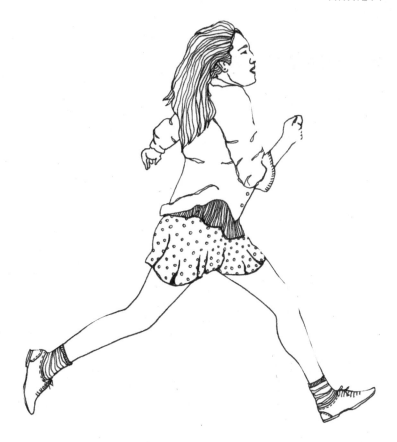

Some other ways people act when they are anxious include:

- Avoiding other people

- Insisting on following an exact routine

- Asking the same questions over and over again

- Pacing up and down

- Hitting out

- Staying near their parents

- Doing the same thing again and again (even though they are not enjoying it)

Do you ever do any of these?

THE ANXIETY LOOP

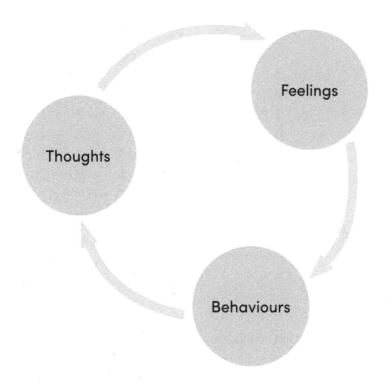

Sometimes people get caught in an anxiety **loop**, **circle** or **cycle** where they have an anxious thought (like 'I can't do this!'), which leads to an anxious feeling (like stress, panic or fear), which leads to an anxious behaviour or act (like hiding in their room). And do you know what hiding in your room leads to? MORE new anxious thoughts, MORE anxious feelings and MORE anxious behaviours, and so on and so on. This loop just keeps going round and round while anxiety keeps getting BIGGER and BIGGER. But never fear – YOU have the power to break out of this loop using the tactics in this book!

WHY DO WE FEEL ANXIETY?

Long ago, in caveman times, humans were in serious danger of being eaten by big animals. To help keep us alive, our body released a hormone called **adrenaline** when we were afraid. Adrenaline raised our blood sugar levels and made our heart beat faster (which made our breathing faster too). This helped us to be stronger and faster so we could either fight the animal or run away really fast. Sometimes all that adrenaline made us freeze (stay really still) which helped us hide and allow danger (like a big bear) to pass by without seeing us. This is called the **flight, fight or freeze** reaction. It has helped the survival of our species. Back then, by fighting or running our bodies used up all that extra adrenaline and so afterwards we would feel back to normal again (if we weren't eaten!).

The problem is that the human body is still acting like we are cavemen. It hasn't caught up with the fact that most of the things that we are worried about these days (like homework, fitting in or leaving our parents) can't actually kill us. The best way to deal with *these* kinds of challenges is to stay calm and figure out solutions logically, not fight or run! But instead, our bodies (still stuck in the caveman days) send out DANGER messages (i.e. too much adrenaline) as if there is a lion in the room trying to eat us. And then because we don't fight or run, all that adrenaline stays in our body causing all kinds of trouble. Not very helpful, is it?

ANXIETY AND THE AUTISM SPECTRUM

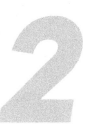

People on the autism spectrum have so many brilliant personality qualities.

- They are honest

- They are direct

- They are responsible

- They have a brilliant sense of right and wrong

- They have great focus

- They are especially good at focusing on the *details* of things

- They like to concentrate on one thing at a time

- They know lots of information about some things

- They often like to do things well and properly

- They care about the world

- They accept people for who they are

- They often don't conform to how people think they should behave or look

- They like things around them to be organised and predictable (happen at the same time and when they are supposed to happen)

However, there can be downsides to some of these great qualities – for example, when:

- People don't do what they say they will

- They are asked to pay attention to lots of different things at the same time

- People don't do the right or fair thing (for example, when a teacher gives the whole class a punishment when only one person did something wrong)

- Things don't turn out perfectly

- People change their minds about plans

- Things don't happen on time

- There are changes to their daily routines

- Things don't stay the same

All of these things can lead to anxiety getting BIGGER (if you let them!).

Other things that people on the autism spectrum have said make anxiety bigger include:

- Homework

- School

- Parties

- Organising themselves (like having all the right things in their bag for school)

- Getting washed and dressed every morning

- Understanding why people do or feel certain things

- Girls on the autism spectrum can find it stressful trying to fit in with 'neurotypicals' (people who aren't on the autism spectrum). They say it can feel like they are wearing a mask or camouflage. They can also feel a lot of pressure to look just right (again to fit in)

- Figuring out the neurotypical rules of things like friendships and school

- Just being around other people, especially when there are lots of them

- When there is too much information coming at them from the world (noises, smells, sights, sounds and things touching them)

Sometimes it is not just one of these things that causes anxiety. Sometimes it is lots of little things throughout the day that they say build and build until their body goes into crisis DANGER mode. This can sometimes mean that while they can manage to stay calm in school, they can have a meltdown over something small once they get home.

And you know what? This world *is* an unpredictable, loud and messy place! No matter how hard you or your parents or your teachers work at making your days predictable, safe and quiet, things will not always go your way. Buses arrive late, tablets run out of battery life, teachers give homework, people tell lies, car alarms go off.

You can't control everything in life and you won't be able to get rid of anxiety altogether (that wouldn't be normal). But remember that you are STRONG, and you CAN control what you THINK, how you FEEL and how you BEHAVE. You CAN learn strategies to help you cope with and manage anxiety and make your days CALMER and HAPPIER, and this book is going to help you do it.

STIMMING
(OR SELF-STIMULATORY BEHAVIOUR)

Of course, lots of people on the spectrum have an inbuilt way to destress – stimming (for example, humming, rocking, making noises, flapping their hands or jumping up and down). People on the autism spectrum have said these things about stimming:

- It helps regulate the sensory information of the world

- It stops them getting overstimulated

- It is like a relief and a release

- It helps prevent an explosion, like the steam being let out of a boiling pot of water

- It reduces tension and helps calm them down

- It is like a bubble of comfort and total relaxation

- It soothes their nervous system

- It feels good

- It is necessary

- It helps them breathe and slow down

Everyone on the spectrum is different. Stimming helps some people concentrate on what is happening around them. Stimming takes some people out of the world around them (it helps them block everything out). Some people don't want to appear different to neurotypicals and so hide their stimming. But lots of other people on the spectrum feel that they shouldn't have to conform to how other people expect them to behave. Especially when they are doing nothing wrong! If stimming helps you block out the world, be careful about when you use it, because sometimes you need to be aware of what is going on around you. Either way, it is a good idea to have a few different tactics to help you relax. If you don't want to stim when other people are looking at you (for example, in certain places like school), you could try to find similar ways of releasing that energy that are less noticeable (like squeezing a stress ball or some of the body exercises in this book).

GETTING HELP

Nobody feels happy all of the time. It is normal to feel different positive and negative emotions during your day, sometimes even at the same time. Feeling anxiety is a part of being human, and it will come and go. But if you are feeling negative emotions like anxiety (or sadness, or anger) ALL of the time, it is a good idea to tell a trusted adult, so that they can help you find ways to be calmer and happier. This might mean talking to someone like a psychologist or a counsellor. It might mean taking medication. Remember: people can't help you unless they know what you are thinking and how you are feeling, and they can't know these things unless YOU let them know.

THINGS YOU CAN DO TO BEAT ANXIETY

GET TO KNOW YOU

This seems a bit weird, doesn't it?

You might be thinking, 'Of course I know me.'

I know what I like (my dog and my iPad) and what I don't like (broccoli and homework).

But actually, we all have stuff going on in our brains and our bodies that we aren't aware of.

Like the thoughts we have when we are stressed (a kind of voice in your head – which is really just you!).

Or how our bodies feel when we are angry or anxious.

You might know you don't like something but do you know why?

Do you know how being on the autism spectrum affects **you**?

Answer these questions to start getting to know you:

- In which places do you feel most relaxed?

- Of all the things you like doing, during which ones are you most relaxed?

- What time of the day do you feel most relaxed?

- With which people do you feel most relaxed?

- What kinds of things do you think about when you are relaxed? What does that 'voice' in your head say?

- How does your body feel when you are relaxed?

- What things do you choose to do when you are relaxed?

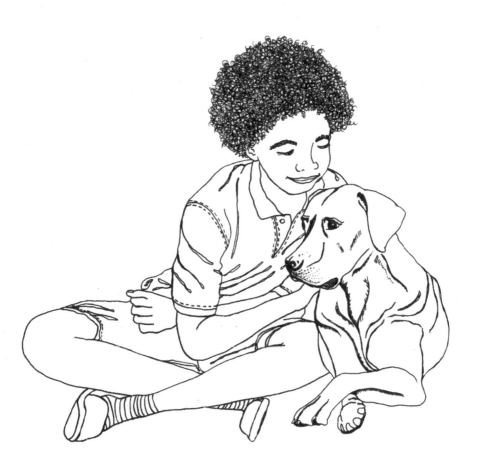

Also:

- In which places do you feel most anxious?

- Of all the things you don't like doing, during which ones do you feel the most anxious?

- What time of the day do you feel most anxious?

- Is there anyone that you feel very anxious when you are around them?

- What kinds of things do you think about when you are anxious? What does that 'voice' in your head say?

- How does your body feel when you are anxious?

- What things do you choose to do when you are anxious?

Write, type or draw pictures of all of your answers. Make them into a list of things, all about YOU.

FINDING IT DIFFICULT TO ANSWER THESE? TRY THIS!

Use a 10-point scale (where 1 is very calm and 10 is anxiety meltdown). Do what you would do on any normal day, but every so often (maybe every half an hour – you can set a timer if it helps) note (1) where you are, (2) what you are doing, (3) who you are with and (4) how anxious you feel on a scale of 1 to 10. At the end of the day or week, look back at all your scores and see where, when and with whom you felt the most anxious. It is a good idea to get a trusted adult to help you with this.

CHANGE WHAT YOU CAN

Look over your list of things all about you.

In this list are things in your life that increase anxiety and things that decrease anxiety.

One of the best things that you can do for a calmer and happier life is to make CHANGES so that you are doing MORE of the things that decrease anxiety and LESS of the things that increase it.

Unfortunately, there are lots of things in life that you will want to change but can't.

For example: school.

Lots of children feel anxious in school and don't want to go.

But they have to because it is the law!

The good news is that even though you still have to go to school, there *are* things about school that you might be able to change.

- If your locker is in a busy hall, you could ask for it to be moved somewhere quieter.

- If you hate having nothing to do at break time, you could ask to do an activity you like, such as playing chess.

- If you don't like the loud noise in the lunchroom, you could ask to eat your lunch somewhere else, or you could wear headphones.

- If music is something that really relaxes you and helps you get through the day, you could ask for scheduled 'music breaks'.

- If your school bag is too heavy, you could ask to have two sets of books, one at home and one at school.

- If there is a lightbulb flickering somewhere that is really bothering you, you could tell a teacher.

- Someone might be bullying you. Telling your parents and teacher means that they can try to do something to stop it. You can also learn ways to deal with it.

Now make two new lists: 'Things I CAN Change' and 'Things I CAN'T Change' (remember they don't *all* have to be about school!).

A trusted adult can help you with this.

A trusted adult can also help you with ideas about how to make these changes happen.

Accepting that you can't change everything, but taking control and changing the things you can, is one of the best ways to beat anxiety!

LEARN ABOUT EMOTIONS (AND TRY NOT TO AVOID THEM)

You are probably not going to like this one!

People on the autism spectrum usually have difficulty learning about emotions.

They feel all the same emotions as everyone else and know other people feel emotions.

But sometimes they have difficulty understanding *why* they or other people feel them.

It can be especially hard when people feel different emotions about the exact same thing!

Sometimes it can be hard even to know just what emotion it is you are feeling.

Because it is hard, people on the autism spectrum can sometimes avoid learning about or talking about emotions.

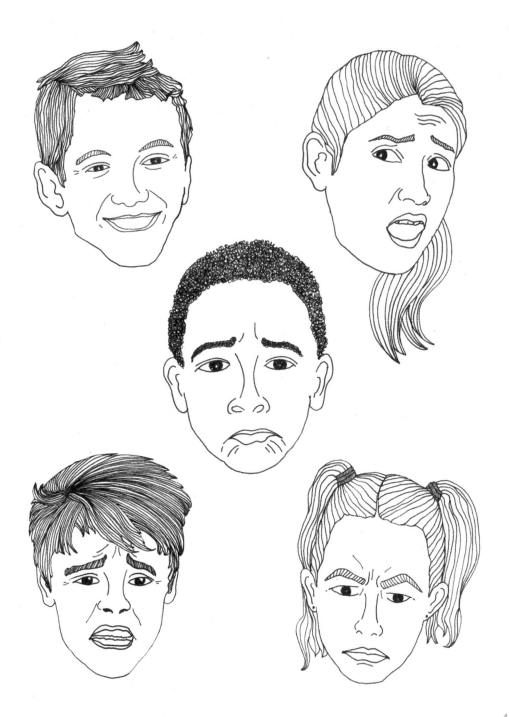

They can sometimes ignore that they are feeling really bad about something and not tell anyone or try to do anything about it.

But the problem with this is that when you ignore or avoid negative feelings like anxiety, they just get worse.

In fact, one of the best ways to have less anxiety in your life is to learn about emotions.

There are lots of ways to do it. Here are a few ideas to get you started:

- Learn about one new emotion every week.

- Don't forget the positive emotions like excitement and love.

- Pretend you are an actor in a movie and you have to show that emotion. What would you look like? What expression would be on your face? What would your body look like? How would you move? How would you feel inside (like how fast would your heart be beating)? What kinds of things would you do or say when feeling that emotion?

- Ask trusted people in your life about their experience of that emotion (try to find someone who likes talking about their emotions – you can ask them politely, 'Would you mind talking to me about your emotions to help me learn?').

- When you are watching a movie or TV show, watch out for different emotions. Look for the body and face 'clues'. Ask a trusted person if you got them correct.

- Watch your favourite TV programme. How many different emotions can you see in one episode? Get someone else to do this at the same time and then compare notes.

EXPRESS YOUR EMOTIONS

Expressing yourself means letting your thoughts and emotions out.

This is usually done by talking, writing, painting, drawing or other forms of art.

It is not a good idea to ignore emotions or keep them 'locked inside' (nothing is really locked, of course) or hidden.

Keeping negative emotions locked up, hidden or ignoring them just makes them worse. FACT.

It is bad for your health and happiness.

It can even give you head aches or stomach aches.

You can express yourself to **let other people know** how you are feeling.

Or you can express yourself **just for you** (for example, writing something and then throwing it away). Even if no one ever sees it, expressing yourself will still be good for you and help reduce anxiety.

Lots of people on the autism spectrum express how they feel about living with autism by writing books or blogs or making videos.

A good one to look up online is Rosie King's Ted Talk, where she talks all about 'how autism freed me to be myself'.

SOME TIPS TO HELP YOU EXPRESS YOUR THOUGHTS AND FEELINGS

- Try different things, like painting, drawing or sculpture.

- Write a song, rap or poem.

- Try typing on a computer, phone or tablet if you find talking difficult.

- If you want your thoughts and feelings to be read, you could write short notes and leave them in a designated place for your parents or teacher to read.

- Have a secret diary or journal where you write about your emotions just for yourself.

- Come up with a code so you can write about your feelings privately.

LOOK AFTER YOUR BODY

One of the absolute best ways that you can reduce anxiety is to look after your body. This means (1) getting enough sleep, (2) eating the right foods, (3) drinking enough water and (4) getting enough exercise. If your body is a machine, these are the four things that are necessary to keep it working well.

Your body gives you signals when it is tired, hungry, thirsty or needs to use up some energy. For example, you might feel a bit dizzy when very hungry, or you might get clumsy when you are tired. But sometimes these signals get a bit messed up and hard to understand, especially when you are on the autism spectrum. For this reason, it is a good idea to get into a routine, where you make sure that you eat, sleep, drink and exercise at around the same time every day. This will stop your body getting too tired, hungry or thirsty and will help prevent anxiety building up. It will also help build up those good HABITS that you read about earlier.

EXERCISE

When you exercise, things called endorphins are released in your body. Endorphins are like natural pain killers which help improve your mood. After exercise, your muscles relax and your heart rate slows down (which is a good thing – heart rates are usually high when you are anxious). Exercise improves your memory. It helps your body fight off diseases. It even helps you sleep better, which also reduces anxiety.

However, there is no point in forcing yourself to do a type of exercise that you hate. You will, I hope, be exercising for the rest of your life: that's a long time to spend on something you're not happy doing.

There are people on the spectrum who are great at group sports, but many find all those people and rules hard to keep up with. For them, sports like running, swimming, boxing or martial arts such as karate can be great. Lots of people on the spectrum love swimming, and say they love the feeling of the deep pressure when their bodies are under the water. Dancing to your favourite music is a great and fun way to improve mood and get some exercise at the same time. Try dancing in your room for a few minutes in the morning before school! Yoga is also a brilliant way to relax, while exercising at the same time, and once you learn some basic yoga techniques you can even do them on your own at home.

FOOD AND WATER

Your body needs enough energy from food to get it through the day. It needs just the right mix of vitamins. It also needs water to keep it hydrated.

Lots of people on the autism spectrum only like certain foods (although lots are lucky enough to like a wide variety of foods). The problem when you don't like certain foods (like fruit or vegetables) or you eat too much of other foods (like high sugar and fat foods) is that your body might not be getting what it needs to stay calm and healthy. Remember that too much food is also bad for your body.

Your body is like a machine – what would happen if instead of putting oil in your car you put in sugary coffee? The car would break down! Your body is like that. If it doesn't get the right kind of foods it will get sick, and you will feel more tired, more anxious and less able to think clearly.

There are some foods that increase anxiety and you should have less of (like caffeine, coffee, tea, chocolate and sugar). But the most important thing is that you are eating mostly healthy food most of the time. A few treats are fine!

Some people even say that foods like turkey, chicken, brown rice, milk, yoghurt, avocados, spinach, tuna and broccoli help with anxiety.

GETTING USED TO NEW FOODS

A good way to get used to a new type of food is to start small, by putting just a tiny bit on your plate. Smell it and touch it but just leave it there. Do this for a week. The next week you could try licking the food before putting it back on your plate. The next week you could take a *tiny* bite. Doing this kind of thing will help you get used to foods you thought you would never eat. You might even surprise yourself by liking them in time.

SLEEP

Lots of people on the autism spectrum find it difficult to sleep, especially when they are worried about something. But the problem is that brains need sleep to recharge. And when they don't recharge, they stop working properly. When your brain is tired, troubles seem a lot worse. It is harder to get the energy to cope with anything, or put effort into changing anything for the better.

Here are some tips for a better night's sleep:

- No screen time for an hour before bed. Your brain thinks the screen light is sunlight, and gets alert as if it is the middle of the day. It is like giving your brain a shot of coffee!

- Try to go to bed at a similar time every night.

- Try to get up at a similar time every morning.

- Have a few nice things you do every night before bed, like having a cup of hot milk and a bath.

- Get exercise during the day.

- Avoid caffeine and sugar.

- Practise some relaxation strategies just before bed (there are lots in this book you can choose from).

- Try not to worry about things once you get into bed. If you really can't stop, try writing your worries down on a note beside the bed and then throwing them away.

- Write a 'To Do' list for the next day before going to sleep, so you can relax that everything is planned for.

LEARN HOW TO DEEP BREATHE

Doing deep breathing is a great tactic because (1) IT WORKS and (2) YOU CAN DO IT ANY TIME, ANYWHERE.

We all breathe all of the time. In and out, in and out.

Most of the time we don't think about or notice it.

When we are relaxed and calm (or asleep) our breathing is slow and steady.

When we are anxious or angry (or exercising), our breathing is fast.

So here is a clever way you can trick your body and mind into being calm.

Just breathe slowly and deeply!

This sends a message from your body to your brain that you are calm.

No danger here. No lions in this room!

Remember: SLOW BREATHING = CALM.

If you are feeling anxious, take three (or more) big, deep, slow breaths in and out.

In through your nose. Out through your mouth.

Pay attention to your breathing while you are doing it.

Feel the air coming in your nose, feel your lungs filling up with air and your tummy getting bigger.

Then feel the air coming out of your mouth, your lungs emptying of air and your tummy getting smaller.

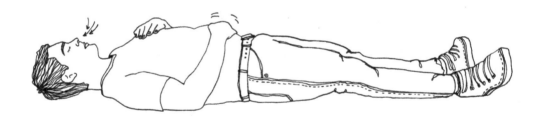

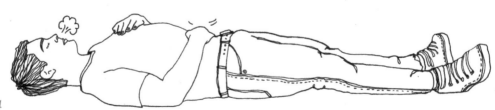

Learning how to deep breathe properly can be a bit tricky. Here are some tips:

- Try lying on the ground with your hands on your stomach so you can feel it going up and down as you breathe.

- Your shoulders and chest area should be relaxed and still when deep breathing. Only your stomach gets bigger or smaller.

- Put a stuffed animal on your stomach and watch as it goes up and down as you breathe (it can be your 'Breathing Buddy').

- Try blowing bubbles. The slow, steady breathing needed for blowing good soap bubbles is just the same as relaxed breathing. Blow the bubble really slowly, and try to get it as big as possible without popping!

- Pretend to be a snake. Take a deep breath in and then hiss slowly like a snake.

- Practise deep breathing when you are calm. It will then make it much easier to do in times of stress.

TOP TIP

Doing deep breathing at the same time as other tactics in this book makes them ALL work even better!

FACE YOUR FEARS

There are some fears that are rational, which means logical, for example when you feel scared or get a bad feeling inside around someone who is mean to you.

However, there are some fears that are *irrational* (they are not logical).

This means that the chance of something bad happening because of this thing is very small.

Some common irrational fears (sometimes called phobias) are of dogs, spiders, bees and flying in airplanes.

The person with the irrational fear might have had a bad experience when they were younger.

They might have been bitten by a bee or they saw a movie about an airplane crash.

Or maybe they just heard a lot of scary things about it, or saw someone else very frightened about that same thing.

Then over the years that fear has got bigger until they are sure that every bee is going to sting them and every plane is going to crash.

And it is true that bees *sometimes* sting (only when they are scared).

It is also true that planes *sometimes* crash (very VERY few of them).

But the chance of either of those things happening to that person is very VERY small.

So what is one of the best ways to make an irrational fear get smaller?

Facing it!

First talk to a trusted adult about it.

Together you can figure out some steps you can take to face your fears really slowly and carefully.

Remember: YOU are in control.

YOU are the one who can face and beat this fear, in your own time.

Here are some examples of some steps you could take to face your fears if you were afraid of dogs:

1. First, look at pictures of dogs.

2. Next, play with a stuffed dog toy.

3. Get a trusted adult to show you with the stuffed animal the ways that dogs like to be petted.

4. Look at videos of happy and calm dogs.

5. After this, visit puppies. You don't even have to go into the same room as them.

6. Pet a puppy being held by someone else.

7. Find someone with a calm and friendly dog. Visit their house with a trusted adult.

8. Be in the same room as the dog.

9. Finally, pet the dog.

Follow these types of steps and see just how **strong you can be** and how **capable you are** at facing and beating your fears!

GIVE ANXIETY A NAME
AND A SHAPE

Giving anxiety a name and a shape means deciding what YOU think anxiety looks like for YOU.

Some people picture anxiety like a cloud above their head getting bigger and darker.

Others think of it like a monster or a zombie from Minecraft taking all of their energy.

Or like an evil plant taking over your mind with its growing tendrils.

Or a computer virus.

Think about a time you felt really anxious or afraid.

Try to remember what it felt like in your body and the kinds of thoughts you had.

Do you have a picture in your head of what it looked like?

Could you give it a name? (Like Dr Dread, The Goblin, Mr Worries or The Cloud of Doom.)

Try drawing a picture of it or writing about it.

You could even write a poem or create a video diary.

Lots of people find it difficult to explain or think about their anxiety.

Don't worry if this tactic takes a while or if you need a bit of grown-up help.

If you can't picture anything, you could use some of the ideas from these pages.

When you use the tactics in this book, try to imagine anxiety (however it looks to you) getting smaller and smaller.

TALK BACK TO ANXIETY

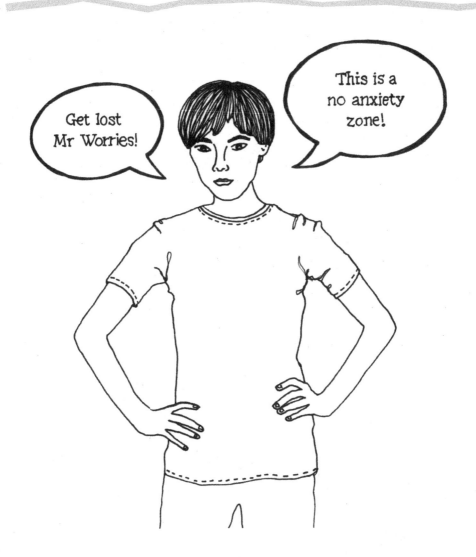

By now you have probably learned a bit about anxiety.

You might have an idea of what anxiety looks like to you.

You might even have given it a name.

Now let's show it who is boss (it's you, by the way!).

There are lots of things you can do to show anxiety you are stronger and cleverer than it.

One of these is to TALK BACK to it.

You know the way in school you are always being told to be polite, especially to teachers?

Well, here you don't have to worry about that *at all*.

When you stop anxious thoughts you stop anxious feelings too.

So next time you notice an anxious thought in your head, try saying one of these to anxiety:

- You lie! I'm not going to listen to you!

- Go away, bug!

- Leave me alone, I don't believe you!

- You're a bully, Dr Dread.

- I'm having a good day today, get lost!

- Back in your box!

Say it strongly and forcefully.

If you are in a place with people around, try saying it in your head.

You could even picture doing something to anxiety, like throwing a pie in its face.

Or you could pretend you are Harry Potter and wave a magic wand at it, making it blow up in smoke or turn into a mouse.

If doing this makes you laugh, even better.

Laughter is one of the BEST ways to beat anxiety.

THROW AWAY ANXIETY

Here is another tactic you can use to make your fears smaller –
throw them away!

This one can be fun.

It can also be good to use if you are on the autism spectrum
because it is VISUAL (which means it is something that you can
actually see in front of you).

People on the autism spectrum are usually GREAT at visual
things.

HOW TO THROW ANXIETY AWAY

- If you are feeling anxious about something, try drawing a picture of it or writing it down on a piece of paper. Then rip up the piece of paper and throw it away!

- Or draw a big red X over the piece of paper.

- Or scribble all over it.

- Stamp on it if you want to! One boy I know loved jumping and climbing and had great fun seeing just how hard and from how high (while still being safe) he could jump on a picture of his fears.

- You could put the pieces of paper away in a special 'anxiety box' or bag.

- One girl I know draws silly underpants and hats on pictures of her fears before throwing them away. This makes her laugh and she says that suddenly anxiety does not seem so serious or powerful any more.

THINK POSITIVE THOUGHTS

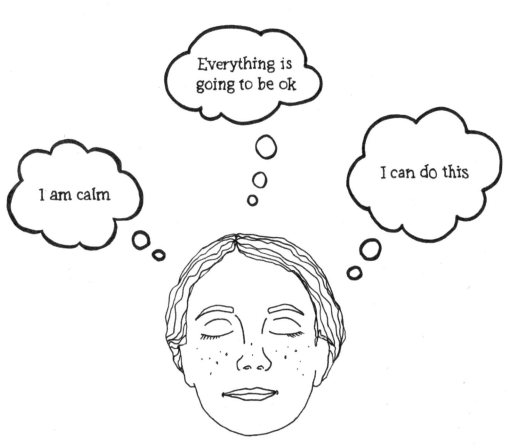

We all think different thoughts all day long.

Some of these thoughts we are aware of.

We know they are there.

We 'hear' them.

Some of these thoughts we are *not* aware of.

We *don't* know they are there.

We *can't* 'hear' them.

When these thoughts are positive and make us feel happy or relaxed, that is great!

But sometimes these thoughts make us feel bad (thoughts like 'I can't do this' or 'Everybody is looking at me').

Sometimes they even make us avoid things we really want to do.

The good news is that research shows that YOU have the power to change negative thoughts to positive thoughts.

Doing this helps your body and mind be more relaxed and happy.

Here are some great positive thoughts:

- I can do this.

- I am a good person.

- The world is full of good things.

- I am strong.

- I am in control.

- All I need to do is try.

- I just haven't figured this out YET.

If you feel anxious in your body, or notice an anxious thought, try saying one of these positive thoughts out loud or in your head.

You might need to say it a few times, or even lots of times.

You can come up with your own calming thoughts or phrases, all the WONDERFUL, POSITIVE things about YOU and how CAPABLE you are.

It is easy to forget about using this tactic, especially when you are feeling anxious.

So it is a good idea to keep a reminder close, like a special bracelet or a list of your positive thoughts in your pocket or phone.

You could even draw a tiny picture on your hand to remind you (since you see your hands a lot during the day).

Try saying your positive thoughts in the morning when you wake up, or before a stressful situation like a party.

The more you say them, the more you will believe them!

IMAGINE RELAXING PICTURES

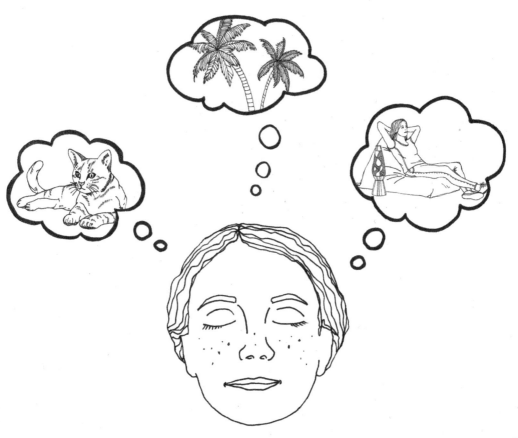

Imagining relaxing pictures is a PROVEN way to lower anxiety.

Using your imagination in this way helps your body and mind to relax.

You might find this one a bit easier than thinking positive *thoughts*, since lots of people on the autism spectrum are great at thinking in pictures.

It's what makes them such amazing engineers, architects and artists.

You can even imagine something like a little movie in your head instead of a picture.

Choosing to change the picture in your head is a bit like changing the channel on your TV.

Here are some examples of things you could imagine.

Try them and see if you feel relaxed when you think about them.

- Your pet

- The sea (with the waves going in and out)

- White clouds floating by in a blue sky

- A special memory you have, for example a family holiday

- Your favourite painting or picture

- Your bedroom

- A battery recharging (going from red to green)

- Bubbles floating up into the air

Even better is if you can really pretend that you are 'in' the picture or movie.

Try to imagine the sounds that you would hear, the smells you would smell, what you might taste and how your body would feel.

If you are ever feeling anxious during the day, try closing your eyes and thinking about your nice, relaxing pictures.

But be careful that you are somewhere safe. This is not a tactic to use when crossing a road!

TRY THIS (BUT ONLY IF YOU LIKE SWIMMING!)

- Close your eyes.

- Pretend that you are at a lovely outdoor swimming pool.

- Imagine the warm sun shining down on you.

- Picture what the water looks like as you get in, sparkling in the sun.

- Imagine what it smells like there – maybe you can smell grass or chlorine.

- Feel the water on your body as you go in.

- Start to swim.

- Feel the water on your arms, legs and body.

- Feel how your body feels under the pressure of the water.

- Hear the water splashing around you.

- Pretend to do a few slow laps up and down the pool (you can be an amazing swimmer in your imagination!).

- Now open your eyes.

How do you feel?

PUT YOUR WORRIES TO THE TEST

This tactic is perfect for people on the autism spectrum because it is all about LOGIC, TRUTH and FACTS, three things they are really good at.

Some people worry and worry about something that *might* happen in the future (for example, being in a car crash).

But they don't *know* it will happen.

Some people go around feeling and thinking like some disaster is about to happen.

But people can't see into the future.

And very few things that happen in life are truly catastrophic.

These worries are not based on FACT.

These people are wasting a lot of time being miserable about something that might NEVER happen.

And most negative events if they do happen turn out to be a LOT less awful than predicted.

Worrying doesn't make a lot of sense, does it?

Also, remember those negative thoughts you read about on page 20?

Thoughts like 'Nobody loves me' or 'I always fail at everything.'

Here is another example of thoughts that are NOT based on FACT.

The person who had the 'Nobody loves me' thought had probably forgotten about their mother, their auntie or a special friend who loves them dearly.

The person who had the 'I always fail at everything' thought had probably forgotten about their medal in Tai Kwan Do or how good they are with computers.

Are you worried about something that *might* happen in the future?

Or do you ever have negative thoughts about yourself?

Learn to think logically instead!

Every time you notice these thoughts or worries, think:

- Is it really true?

- Is there evidence that it is NOT true?

- What are the FACTS?

REMEMBER

It is IMPOSSIBLE to stop a bad thing happening by worrying about it.

BE MINDFUL

Being mindful means being AWARE.

It means noticing your thoughts, feelings, body sensations, and anything that is around you RIGHT NOW.

It is all about staying PRESENT (in the HERE and NOW), instead of worrying about something that might happen in the future.

It is also all about calmly accepting the thoughts and feelings you are having right now.

Focusing on the HERE and NOW helps reduce anxiety. FACT.

As someone on the autism spectrum, you are probably great at being mindful at times, like when you are really aware of the noises, sights and smells around you.

You probably already know the peace and happiness that comes with concentrating on doing just one thing.

However, Mindfulness tactics are NOT the best tactic to use when you are overwhelmed by sensory information (sights, sounds, smells, noises), for example in a busy shopping centre.

In these moments you probably need to be a bit LESS aware of everything around you.

But Mindfulness tactics *are* good to use when you are worrying about what might happen in the future.

Or if you are having negative thoughts that are making you feel bad.

That is because BEING MINDFUL takes you away from those thoughts, and helps you concentrate instead on the wonderful things around you.

They bring you back into REALITY.

THREE WAYS TO BE MINDFUL DURING YOUR DAY

1. Go for a 'noticing walk'. Pay attention to what you can see, hear, feel and smell. If your mind starts thinking about other things, just gently bring it back to whatever is actually going on around you.

2. If you notice negative thoughts, try not to be angry, ignore them or try to get rid of them (remember, ignoring emotions just makes them worse!). Instead, just notice them. Pretend to say 'Hi' to them, if that doesn't feel too silly. Notice how anxiety feels in your body, and remember that **it is just a feeling, it is not your fault**, and **it will go away**.

3. Or instead, when you feel them, concentrate instead on your five senses:

    *   What can I feel?
    *   What can I smell?
    *   What can I taste?
    *   What can I hear?
    *   What can I see?

Doing this will help you return back to reality again.

MEDITATE

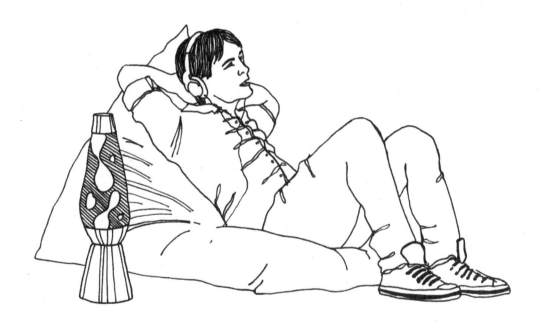

Being mindful and meditation are both proven ways to help yourself be calmer and healthier.

But they are actually quite different.

Being MINDFUL is all about being AWARE of the world around you.

MEDITATION is all about taking yourself OUT of the world by focusing on one thought, chant, object or sound.

Meditation is like a charger for the brain.

If you do it in the morning, it can give you energy.

If you do it at night time, it can clear your head and help you get to sleep more easily.

Meditation can even help you concentrate better in school or on homework.

It can also help prevent build-ups of anxiety that lead to meltdown.

There are lots of different ways to meditate.

You might need to try a few different types before finding the one that works for you.

There are plenty of meditation videos, apps and CDs that you can try.

Meditation can feel uncomfortable at first.

It can take a while to get used to it.

TIPS TO GET YOU STARTED

- Go to a safe and quiet place.

- Turn off phones, tablets and computers.

- Set a timer for 1 or 2 minutes.

- Get into a comfortable position.

- Close your eyes.

- Remain still and quiet.

- Concentrate on your breathing going in and out (see page 53 for some tips), or think of a picture, or repeat one word or phrase or sound (like 'OM') over and over in your head.

- If your mind starts thinking about other things, just gently bring it back to what you have decided to concentrate on. Don't get cross or frustrated when this happens – it is normal and you will do it less with practice.

- Keep concentrating on the one thing while breathing slowly in and out.

- When the timer goes off, stop meditating.

DAILY RELAXING TIME

This is probably the easiest tactic in the whole book!

All you have to do is sit and relax in a special relaxing place.

It doesn't have to be a whole room – it could be a corner in a room.

Some people like this space to be covered, like a tent or fort.

Make sure it is comfy to sit in – you could try using a beanbag or big cushions.

You might like to have a few reminders of nature there, like a nice plant or some pebbles from the beach.

Put up posters or pictures of things that make you feel relaxed when you look at them.

Nice lighting (for example, fairy lights or a special lamp) can also help.

While sitting in your relaxing space you don't have to meditate or be mindful or do any of the other tactics in this book (although if you wanted to that would be extra great!).

You can do absolutely nothing if you want to.

Or you can listen to music, think about something you are really interested in or pet your dog.

Basically, do anything you find relaxing.

YOU CAN USE THIS RELAXING SPACE IN A FEW DIFFERENT WAYS

- You could go there at least once a day to prevent build-ups of anxiety.

- You could go there after times when you are around a lot of people and noise (like the supermarket or school) to help you wind down.

- You could go there if you feel anxiety or other negative emotions in your body.

It is not always possible for lots of reasons, but try asking for a special relaxing place in your school or classroom if you think this is something that would help you.

WHOLE BODY RELAXATION

This is one great way to relax your body, which also helps relax your mind.

If you are in a safe space, you can lie down on the floor to do it but you don't have to.

You can also just sit somewhere comfortable.

You can even do it sitting in class.

All it involves is tensing (or squeezing) certain parts of your body for a few seconds, and then relaxing them.

You can start at your toes if you want.

Tense your toes – really squeeze them hard for a few seconds.

Then relax them.

Next, make your legs tense. You can squeeze them together or make them go really straight and stiff. Then relax them.

Tense your stomach muscles, then relax them.

Now tense your arms. Squeeze them against your sides or out straight. Then relax them.

Now, squeeze your hands into fists (you can pretend you are squeezing something in your hand). Then relax them.

Bring your shoulders up really high as if you want them to touch your ears. Then relax them.

You can even squish up your face really tight for a few seconds. Then relax it.

It doesn't really matter what order you tense and relax your body parts in, but it is probably helpful to start at one end of your body and work your way through to the other end.

When you are finished, try to relax your body so that all of your muscles are as loose as possible.

Pretend your body is made of jelly or you are a floppy octopus.

THREE WAYS YOUR HANDS AND ARMS CAN HELP YOU RELAX

Here are three more great ways that you can use your body to relax.

You can do these any time, anywhere.

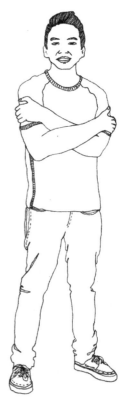

1. **Give yourself a hug.**
    Squeeze firmly. Hold it
    for around 10 seconds.

2. **Massage your arm.** This means squeezing one arm with the hand of your other arm. Start at the top or the bottom of your arm. Squeeze a little bit (whatever is comfortable for you), then move up a little bit and squeeze again. Keep going until you reach the end of your arm. Now go the other way. When you have gone up and down one arm, do the other one.

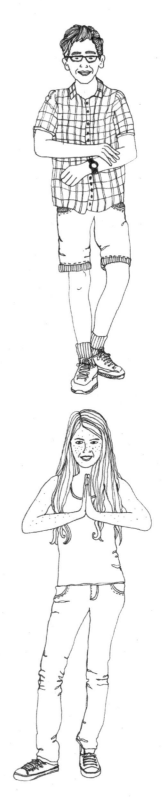

3. **Push your hands together.** Push and hold them like that for around 10 seconds. Then relax.

Try deep breathing at the same time to make these work even better!

HAVE A SIGNAL

When you are feeling anxious (or other strong emotions) it can be hard to use your words to tell people what you need.

This is the same for everyone, but can be even harder when you are on the autism spectrum.

For this reason, it is a good idea to have a SIGNAL (that doesn't involve words) that tells people when you are really anxious.

Examples of signals:

- Rubbing your ear

- Tapping your nose

- Putting your hand on your head

When you use YOUR signal, you are telling people that you are overwhelmed or need a break.

If you don't want everyone knowing you are getting overwhelmed, a signal can get you out of the situations without anyone else noticing.

You can choose who you want to share your signal with.

You can keep it like a secret code between you and other trusted people.

Or you can choose to tell everyone your signal. It is your decision.

Your signal can also mean different things, like:

- I need time alone.

- I need my headphones.

- I need to go for a walk.

- I need you to stop asking me questions.

TRY THIS!

If you want to go to a school disco but are afraid you will get overwhelmed with the lights and noise, make up a secret signal between you and a friend which means that you need someone to go outside with you for a few minutes.

HERE'S YOUR SIGNAL TO DO LIST

1. Come up with a signal.

2. Decide what exactly your signal means (what you want to happen when you make that signal).

3. Decide who you want to tell.

4. Tell them.

5. Practise using it (like you would a fire drill even when there is no fire).

DEALING WITH SENSORY OVERLOAD

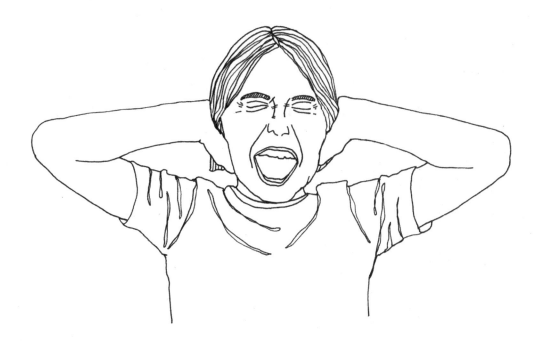

The world can be a busy, noisy place.

Places like shopping centres are especially so.

There could be bright lights, music playing, people talking, people bumping into you by accident, beeping noises, babies crying and the smell of different perfumes going on around you all at the SAME TIME.

Lots of people on the autism spectrum say that this can be TOO MUCH SENSORY INFORMATION.

They say that sometimes all of this information causes SENSORY OVERLOAD.

It is a REALLY good idea to tell people how you feel in these places.

You probably want to avoid them altogether.

But unfortunately there will be times you have to go into them (like if your parents need to buy food and can't leave you at home alone).

So for those times, here are some tips to help stay calm.

Most of them are about distracting yourself and helping to block out at least some of the sensory information from around you:

- Have a plan.

- Find out how long you will be in the place so you will know when the end point will be (but remember that real life doesn't stick to exact schedules).

- Remind yourself that it will not last forever.

- Have a signal to let who you are with know that it has become too much (see page 88).

- Bring something to hold or feel (maybe a favourite scarf, a gel pack or a sensory ball).

- Bring something special to you (like a special toy).

- Wear headphones – either for music or special noise-cancelling headphones.

- Download relaxing music on your phone or tablet to listen to when out.

- Bring a note with reminders about your calming tactics.

- Count to 10 slowly in your head.

- Concentrate on breathing deeply and slowly (see page 53).

- Think positive thoughts (see page 66).

- Imagine relaxing pictures (see page 69).

- Think about things you love and are interested in.

- Try the three hand and arm tactics (see page 86).

- If you love swimming but hate the noise in swimming pool buildings, get waterproof wireless headphones and listen to music.

- If you have a dog, try bringing him with you on a lead. Keeping your focus on him, petting or talking to him will help.

DEALING WITH PANIC ATTACKS

Sometimes, some people get so overwhelmed by anxiety that they have what is called a panic attack.

When this happens their heart starts beating really fast, they feel dizzy and they might have pains in their chest.

Their fingers or toes might feel numb.

They might feel like they can't move their body.

People can have panic attacks not just because of what is going on around them (the sensory overload you read about already), but also what is going on in their head.

They happen because their worries get TOO BIG.

And their bodies react as if there is a tiger in the room and they need to fight, run or freeze.

Panic attacks last about 10–15 minutes but can feel longer.

They are quite common – lots of people have them.

They are also harmless.

You can't die from a panic attack.

It is very important to remember this because getting panicked about having a panic attack just makes everything worse.

If you get panic attacks, the BEST thing to do is work on all of the things in this book and prevent them happening in the first place.

But if you are in the middle of one, the BEST tactic is to BREATHE DEEPLY AND SLOWLY (see page 53).

Keep deep breathing until your body has calmed down.

Try saying the word RELAX in your head or out loud while you breathe.

Try doing the whole body relaxation strategy on page 84.

Picture the place that you are happiest, or imagine your other relaxing pictures.

Say things to yourself like:

- This will pass.

- This is normal.

- Nothing bad is going to happen to me.

- I am strong.

- I will get through this.

You will be calm again soon, no harm done.

PRACTISE BEING GRATEFUL

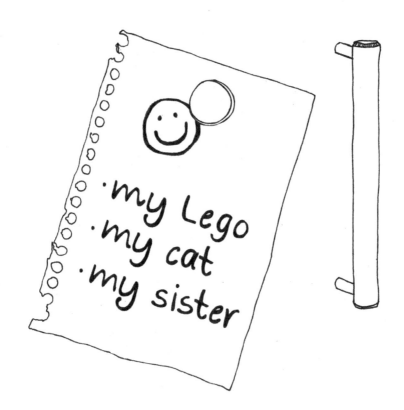

Sometimes life can be difficult.

Bad things can happen.

People can be mean.

Sadness, anger and anxiety are a part of life.

But life can also be wonderful.

Great things happen.

People can be kind.

Happiness, joy and peace are also a part of life.

Being grateful does not mean ignoring the bad things.

But it does mean feeling *thankful for* or *appreciating* the good things.

Being grateful is a skill that you get better at the more you practise.

Learning to be grateful has been proven to make people happier and calmer.

Make a list of the things that you are grateful for.

Your list could include having a great bedroom, a computer, a funny dog, a kind teacher, a medal in maths, something that you are really good at or a hobby that you love doing.

Put your list somewhere you see every day (like your fridge) or type it into your phone.

Of course, your list will change over time.

Make being grateful part of your daily routine.

Look at your list every morning.

If worry tries to take over your thoughts during the day, remind yourself of your list.

Look at it again last thing before sleep.

Remember that the world is full of amazing things.

Don't let anxiety make you miss out on them!

EXTRA INFORMATION FOR ADULTS

INFORMATION FOR PARENTS AND PROFESSIONALS

The information presented and tactics chosen for this book take into account the unique and varied strengths and challenges of young people on the autism spectrum. They are solution focused, grounded in clinical observations (tactics that I have found to be successful with my clients on the autism spectrum) and based on the most up-to-date research (including the Positive Psychology, Cognitive Behavioural Therapy and Mindfulness traditions). They are also written in a format and style that is designed specifically to be accessible to young people on the spectrum.

There are lots of ways that you can support children and teenagers on the spectrum to develop life-long coping skills to manage anxiety.

The first step will be to help the young person recognise and understand anxiety, including how it affects their thoughts, bodies and actions. Knowledge is power. Talking about anxiety (in a calm and factual manner) will not make it worse.

The next step will be helping them to understand themselves, including how being on the autism spectrum affects them and their interactions with the world. A positive attitude towards difference and neurodiversity is of course a given.

The next issue is does the young person *want* to change? To take on board the tactics in this book and really make them work *for them*, the young person will need to see and understand the benefits of their hard work. If they do not want to change at this time, it is worth showing them all the great things they will be able to do with a few tactics under their belt, for example going to that comic book conference or the same parties as their sister.

But in addition to the young person learning skills, the important adults in their lives also need to be aware of how **they react** to the young person's anxiety. Remember that how you as an adult react has the power either to increase or decrease a young person's anxiety. Be very careful of the messages you give them. Take, for example, a father who when his daughter becomes anxious in a playground immediately picks her up and takes her hurriedly home. Does this reaction tell his daughter that she is capable of overcoming her anxiety and making her own decisions? Or does it tell her that she needs minding and protection from a dangerous world that she can't handle or cope with by herself? What do you think this girl is most likely to do next time she feels anxious? The best way to respond to a young person's anxiety is with a firm and loving calmness, and by helping them come up with their own solutions to problems, even if this means sometimes making mistakes. They need to get the message from you that (1) **they are capable** and (2) **the world is a safe place** (at least most of the time).

Important adults also need to **model** for the young person healthy ways of managing anxiety and other strong negative emotions. This will include how you react on a day-to-day basis to irritations (for example, trying to stay calm when stuck in traffic by putting on relaxing music). It will also include normalising worry and using the tactics in this book yourself. Also important will be modelling more general self-care, including taking time for your own interests, meeting friends and looking after your own mental and physical health. If you are finding it difficult to respond to a young person's distress in a calm and supportive manner, consider seeking additional support for yourself from a mental health professional. Think of looking after yourself like needing to put your own oxygen mask on first on an airplane. Sometimes you have to look after yourself first in order to help someone else.

You might also need to consider accessing professional support from a mental health professional for the young person if difficulties with anxiety persist, but do try to ensure that they are fully qualified and have experience with young people on the autism spectrum.

HOW TO REACT IF YOUR CHILD IS
HAVING A PANIC ATTACK

Most importantly, stay calm. Your child will notice your
calm voice and body language and react well to this. Be
confident and reassuring. Keep your sentences short
and simple (if you have pictures to represent what you
are saying even better). Explain to them that everything
is OK. Remind them that what they are going through is
common and will be over soon. Help them leave the
situation and go somewhere quiet and relaxing. Help
them to concentrate on slow, deep breathing and
other simple relaxation techniques like the whole body
relaxation on page 84. Stay with them until they have
calmed down.

This book contains just a short selection of the many tactics that
can help young people with anxiety. Here are a few more ideas
and recommendations:

- Deep pressure and massage is a tactic that many parents
  of children on the spectrum report to be effective, giving
  their children a deep-pressure massage before bed, and
  after school or other stressful situations.

- Coping Cards could be made up, each one containing
  a picture or explanation of a strategy from this book.

These can be shown to the child as reminders when out and about.

- Spending time with animals is a proven way to improve mood and reduce anxiety, and many people on the spectrum have spoken about their love for and affinity with animals. Pets can be great companions and help ease loneliness. Having a dog is also a great way of encouraging exercise and being outside in nature (both of which are also proven to increase mood and reduce anxiety). If you can't have a pet at the moment, just watching funny dog and cat videos has been shown to have benefits to mood.

- Bring relaxation practices (for example, meditation, Mindfulness or yoga) into your daily lives as a family. If you are a teacher, incorporate relaxation into daily teaching practices. Research shows that daily meditation in class can increase attention and productivity and decrease challenging behaviours. The recommended resources section contains books with lots of activities that can be used. However, you can find plenty of free child and teen meditations and recommendations online.

- Try using the young person's special interest to make the tactics in this book more meaningful for them. For example, anxiety could be personified as one of the baddies from Minecraft and the tactics could be described as tools to keep the baddies away.

- There are many more excellent Cognitive Behavioural Therapy (CBT) strategies (in particular cognitive strategies) that are not included in this book because of the high level of language and metacognitive skills required. However, if a young person has good language skills and can think about their thinking, it may be worthwhile pursuing these cognitive tactics in more depth, for example by accessing CBT from a mental health professional or using workbooks with a CBT focus (for example, *Starving the Anxiety Gremlin* or *The Anxiety Workbook for Teens*: see pages 108–109 for full reference details).

- Try different relaxation, CBT, meditation or Mindfulness apps with the young person, many of which are free.

- Sports psychologists have found that the best thing to do with pre-game anxiety is not to reduce it but to **reframe** it as **excitement**. This helps the athletes perform at their best. If you know a child who is experiencing anxiety before things like concerts or games, try this reframing technique. A sample script might be 'It's normal to be nervous before a match. But you know those feelings in your stomach? Those feelings are also excitement. They are going to help you do really well in this match!'

- Of course, beyond CBT there are other therapetic approaches that can help reduce anxiety. Research suggests that accessing a fully qualified, experienced professional with whom the young person has a good therapeutic relationship may predict positive outcomes.

IMPORTANT NOTE ABOUT FACING YOUR FEARS

All young people need to learn that the more you avoid things you find scary, the worse they get. And that a great tactic to stop phobias or other irrational fears is to slowly desensitise yourself to them, that is, gradually facing your fears. However, many children on the spectrum experience genuine pain and discomfort in some situations because of sensory and other issues and forcing exposure to them is unethical and cruel. Also, of course there will be some situations where the young person has good reason to be afraid (for example, they might be afraid of going into school because they are being bullied) but finds it difficult to explain due to language difficulties associated with being on the spectrum. Getting this right will be a delicate balancing act and requires you knowing the child well. Exposure should be very gradual and the child should not be in significant distress at any stage.

RECOMMENDED READING AND RESOURCES FOR PARENTS AND PROFESSIONALS

The Anxiety Workbook for Teens: Activities to Help You Deal with Anxiety and Worry by Lisa M. Schab (2008) New Harbinger

Been There. Done That. Try This! An Aspie's Guide to Life on Earth edited by Tony Attwood, Craig R. Evans and Anita Lesko (2014) Jessica Kingsley Publishers

The Feelings Book (Revised): The Care and Keeping of Your Emotions by Linda Madison (2013) American Girl Publishers

Get Out of Your Mind and Into Your Life for Teens: A Guide to Living an Extraordinary Life by Joseph Ciarrochi, Louise L. Hayes, Ann Bailey and Stephen C. Hayes (2012) New Harbinger

How to Be a Superhero Called Self-Control: Super Powers to Help Younger Children to Regulate Their Emotions and Senses by Lauren Brukner (2015) Jessica Kingsley Publishers

The Kid's Guide to Staying Awesome and in Control: Simple Stuff to Help Children Regulate Their Emotions and Senses by Lauren Brukner (2014) Jessica Kingsley Publishers

M in the Middle: Secret Crushes, Mega-Colossal Anxiety and the People's Republic of Autism by The Students of Limpsfield Grange School and Vicki Martin (2016) Jessica Kingsley Publishers

Relax by Catherine O'Neill (1993) Child's Play International

The *Relax Kids* series of books by Marneta Viegas, O Books

Sitting Still Like a Frog: Mindfulness Exercises for Kids and Their Parents by Eline Snel (2014) Shambhala Publications

Starving the Anxiety Gremlin: A Cognitive Behavioural Therapy Workbook on Anxiety Management for Young People by Kate Collins-Donnelly (2013) Jessica Kingsley Publishers

What to Do When You Worry Too Much: A Kid's Guide to Overcoming Anxiety by Dawn Huebner (2002) Magination Press/American Psychological Association

Davida Hartman is a Director and Senior Educational Psychologist at The Children's Clinic, Dublin, providing child and educational psychology services to children 0–18. She is a lecturer and trainer in the area of autism, and has been working with children and adolescents on the autism spectrum for 16 years in the capacity of a psychologist and a teacher. Davida received her undergraduate degree in Psychology from Trinity College Dublin and her MA in Educational Psychology from University College Dublin. She is a Chartered Psychologist with the Psychological Society of Ireland (PSI). Her website can be visited at www.thechildrensclinic.ie.